NATURAL HIGH BLOOD PRESSURE TREATMENT

DR MIRIAM KINAI

ISBN: 1490489096

ISBN-13: 978-1490489094

CONTENTS

ACKNOWLEDGMENTS

I would like to express my sincere gratitude to everyone who contributed in one way or another to the development of this publication.

I would especially like to thank http://www.zazzle.com/ChristianArtGifts for their photographs.

1

DIET THERAPY

Dietary modifications that you can institute to lower high blood pressure naturally include:

1.

Dietary Approaches to Stop Hypertension (DASH)

DASH is a scientifically proven method of lowering high blood pressure by modifying your diet. Study participants who followed the DASH diet were able to lower their high blood pressure by up to 14mm Hg in a few weeks.

DASH recommendations include eating:

7-8 servings of grain each day in which 1 serving is 1 slice of bread or ½ cup of cooked pasta, rice or 1 oz (30 grams) dry cereal

4-5 servings of vegetables each day in which 1 serving is 1 cup of raw leafy vegetables or ½ cup of raw cut-up vegetables or ½ cup of cooked vegetables or ½ cup vegetable juice

4-5 servings of fruit each day in which 1 serving is 1 medium sized fruit or 1 cup of raw fruit or ½ cup of cooked fruit or ½ cup of fresh, frozen, canned fruit or ½ cup of fruit juice or ¼ cup of dried fruit

2-3 servings of low fat or fat free dairy products each day in which 1 serving is 1 cup (8 oz or 240 ml) of milk or 1 cup (8 oz or 240 ml) of yogurt or 1 ½ oz (45 grams) of cheese

2 servings of meat, fish, or poultry each day in which 1 serving is 3 oz (90 grams) of cooked meat, fish, poultry or 3 oz (90 grams) of tofu

2-3 servings of fats and oils each day in which 1 serving is 1 teaspoon of olive oil, margarine, mayonnaise or 1 tablespoon regular salad dressing or 2 tablespoons of low fat salad dressing

4-5 servings of nuts, seeds, and dry beans each week in which 1 serving of nuts is 1/3 cup (1.5 oz) of nuts or 2 tablespoons (1/2 oz or 15 grams) seeds or 2 tablespoons peanut butter or ½ cup dry beans, peas

4 servings of sweets each week in which 1 serving is 1 tablespoon sugar or 1 tablespoon jam, jelly or 1 cup lemonade or ½ cup sorbet

***

2.

DASH-Sodium

The DASH-Sodium is a modified DASH diet which recommends reducing your sodium intake to 1500 mg a day which is roughly equivalent to 2/3 teaspoon of salt. This DASH-Sodium has also been shown to lower high blood pressure.

Therefore reduce your salt intake and avoid high sodium foods like potato crisps, bacon and processed meats.

***

3.

Eat Potassium Rich Foods

Increasing your intake of potassium rich foods can help you lower high blood pressure naturally. Perfect examples of potassium rich foods include bananas, orange juice, spinach and tomato juice.

If you have kidney disease consult your doctor before increasing your intake of potassium rich foods. In addition, understand that increasing your intake of potassium rich foods should go hand in hand with reducing your intake of sodium rich foods.

***

4.

Eat Calcium Rich Foods

Increasing your intake of calcium and magnesium rich foods like milk, yoghurt, cheese and green leafy vegetables can lower blood pressure.

***

5.

Eat Vitamin C Rich Foods

Increasing your intake of Vitamin C rich foods like oranges, grapefruits, tangerines, lemons and other citrus fruits can also help lower high blood pressure.

***

6.

Reduce Caffeine Intake

Since drinking beverages with caffeine like coffee can raise your blood pressure, reduce your intake of caffeinated beverages.

***

DASH Meal Plan

The following is a simplified DASH meal plan:

Breakfast: 2 servings grain, 1 serving fats, 1 serving fruits, 1 diary

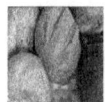 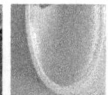 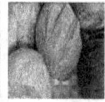 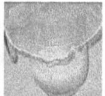

Mid morning snack: 1 serving grain, 1 serving low fat dairy, 1 serving fruits, 1 serving nuts (snack on nuts on 5 days per week)

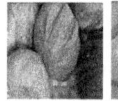 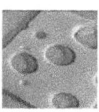 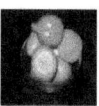 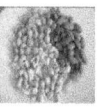

Lunch: 4 servings grain, 1 serving fats, 1 beef, chicken or fish, 2 servings vegetables, 1 serving fruit

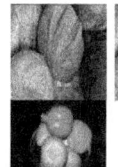 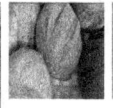 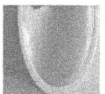 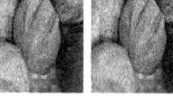 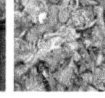 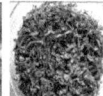 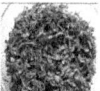

Mid afternoon snack: 2 servings fruit, 1 serving low fat dairy

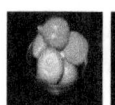 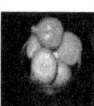 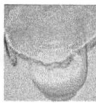

Dinner: 3 servings grain, 1 serving fats, 1 chicken, beef or fish, 3 serving vegetables, 1 serving dessert (for only 4 days per week)

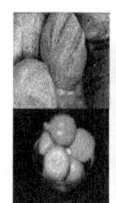 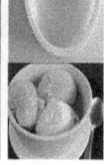 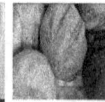 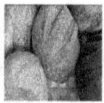 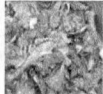 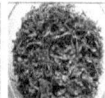 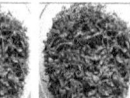 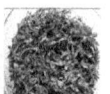

* * * * *

2

SUPPLEMENTS

Supplements that can help lower high blood pressure include:

1.

CoEnzyme Q10

Studies have shown that taking CoEnzyme Q10 can lower high blood pressure. In one study in which the participants where taking 60 mg of CoEnzyme Q10 twice a day, their blood pressure was reduced by over 15mmHg.

***

2.

Folic Acid

Folic acid, which is one of the B complex vitamins, is thought to lower high blood pressure by lowering homocysteine levels.

***

3.

Omega 3 Fatty Acids

Fish oil supplements which contain DHA (docohexaenoic acid) and EPA (eicosapentaenoic acid) have been shown to reduce high blood pressure in persons with mild hypertension.

***

4.

Garlic

Garlic has been shown to be effective in lowering high blood pressure and garlic supplements can be taken if one cannot tolerate the odor of natural garlic cloves.

***

5.

L-arginine and L-taurine

L-arginine and L-taurine, which are amino acids, are also thought to help lower blood pressure.

***

6.

Daily Multivitamin

A multi-vitamin, multi-mineral supplement that is well balanced and that contains calcium, magnesium, vitamin C, and the B complex vitamins in their daily recommended values should be taken every day.

* * * * *

3

HERBS

Herbs that may be beneficial for the management of high blood pressure include:

1.

Hawthorn Berry

Hawthorn has been used for a long time by herbalists to lower high blood pressure. Their claims were proven in a study conducted in Reading, UK in which participants who were taking 1200 mg of hawthorn extract each day were found to have lower blood pressures at the end of the study.

***

2.

Garlic

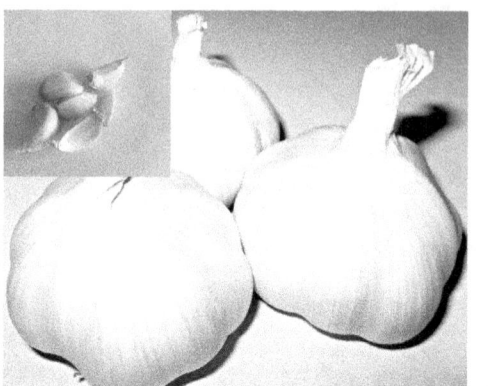

Garlic contains allicin which has blood pressure lowering properties. In a study done at the *Clinical Research Center of New Orleans* patients who had severe hypertension were noted to have reduced blood pressure on taking a garlic preparation with 1.3 % allicin.

A previous study demonstrated that fresh garlic was more potent in protecting the heart than processed garlic. Therefore, swallow the cloves raw or add them to your cooked dishes. You can also squeeze the garlic cloves and drink the fresh juice.

* * * * *

4

ESSENTIAL OILS

Aromatherapy is the use of essential oils for their healing benefits. Each essential oil has a unique scent and effect on the mind and body.

Though aromatherapy has not been proven to cure hypertension, some essential oils are known to lower blood pressure and they can be used by persons with hypertension.

Essential oils which have mentally relaxing properties can also be used since stress raises blood pressure.

Essential oils that are used to manage hypertension include lavender, marjoram, clary sage, and ylang ylang.

Clary Sage Essential Oil

Botanical name: Salvia sclarea

Perfumery Note: Top note

Clary Sage Essential Oil Safety Information

1. Do not use it during pregnancy.

2. Do not use it if you are drinking alcohol or driving.

3. Do not use if if you have endometriosis, ovarian cysts, uterine cysts, breast cancer or you are at high risk for developing breast cancer as it may have an "estrogen-like" effect on the body.

4. Preparations with a high concentration of clary sage can result in a narcotic effect. Therefore, avoid using more than 0.8% concentrations.

5. Clary sage can also cause headaches.

***

Lavender Essential Oil

Botanical name: Lavendula officinalis

Perfumery Note: Middle note

Lavender Essential Oil Safety Information

1. Do not use it in pregnancy especially the first 3 months.

2. Do not use it if you are breastfeeding.

3. Do not use it on young children as it may cause breast development in boys (gynaecomastia) and girls (pre-pubescent breast development).

4. Avoid it if you have low blood pressure as you may feel drowsy after using it.

***

Marjoram Essential Oil

Botanical name: Origanum marjorana

Perfumery Note: Middle note

Marjoram Essential Oil Safety Information

1. Do not use it if you have low blood pressure.

2. Do not use it if you are pregnant.

***

Ylang Ylang Essential Oil

Botanical name: Cananga odorata

Perfumery Note: Base note

Ylang Ylang Essential Oil Safety Information

1. Avoid it if you have low blood pressure.

2. Avoid using it if you have sensitive or damaged skin.

3. Preparations with a high concentration of ylang ylang can cause headaches and nausea. Therefore, avoid using more than 1% concentrations.

***

Using Essential Oils for High Blood Pressure

The first step in using essential oils to manage high blood pressure is to do a patch test for each of the essential oils that you want to use.

To do this, simply apply the essential oil that has been diluted with a carrier oil on the inner aspect of your elbow, bandage it and wait for 24 hours to see if you will develop rashes or itchiness or swelling or any other sign of an allergic reaction. If you do, do not use that essential oil.

The second step is to create the essential oil blend that you will use to manage hypertension. A simple "Anti-Hypertension Blend" can be made by mixing 10 drops of Ylang ylang essential oil, 20 drops of lavender essential oil, 20 drops of Marjoram essential oil and 30 drops of Clary sage essential oil in a dark bottle.

We will refer to this mixture as "Anti-Hypertension Blend" in our recipes. Therefore, if the recipe says, "Add 12 drops of the Anti-Hypertension Blend", you simply add 12 drops of this mixture.

If you just want to buy one aromatherapy oil to experiment with, I would recommend marjoram essential oil. Likewise, if the recipe says, "Add 12 drops of the Anti-Hypertension Blend", you simply add 12 drops of marjoram essential oil.

Aromatherapy Bath.

Create a healing bath by dispersing 12 drops of the "Anti-Hypertension Blend" in your warm bath water. You can also mix the essential oils with milk to help them disperse.

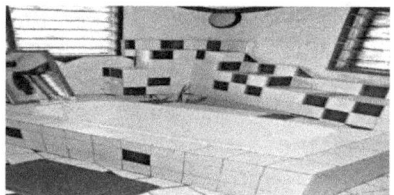

Bath Gel.

Add 50 drops (2.5 ml or ½ teaspoons) of the "Anti-Hypertension Blend" to one cup (8 oz or 250 ml) of unscented bath gel or liquid soap to create a healing bath gel.

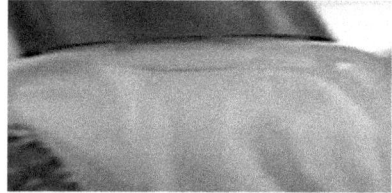

Bath Salts.

Mix 2 cups of Epsom salts, 1 cup of sea salt and 1 cup of baking soda. Add 50 drops (2.5 ml) of the "Anti-Hypertension Blend" and a few drops of food coloring (optional). Add one cup of this mixture to your warm bath water for a healing invigorating soak.

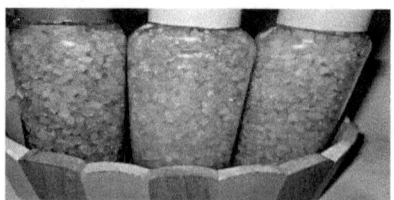

Bath Tea.

Mix 2 cups of lavender flowers with 15 drops of the "Anti-Hypertension Blend" and 1 cup of sea salt. Put the mixture in an air tight jar or you can add a scoopful of the mixture into a cotton bath tea bag and store the filled bath tea bags in the air tight jar.

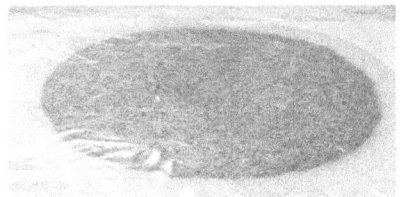

Body Lotion.

Heat 6 oz or 190 ml of sweet almond oil and 1.5 oz or 45 grams of grated beeswax in a double boiler or water bath until the beeswax melts and mixes completely with the vegetable oils. Remove the mixture from the heat and let it cool completely. Put 8 oz or 250 ml water in a blender and with the blender on high speed, slowly pour in the cooled vegetable oil and beeswax mixture. Blend until the mixture emulsifies and forms a thick, creamy lotion. Add 10-20 drops of the "Anti-Hypertension Blend" drop by drop as you blend until you get your required scent. Pour your lotion in a glass jar.

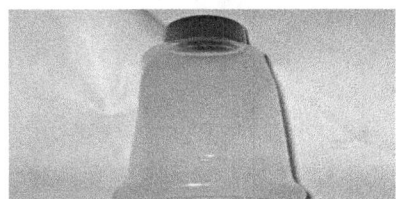

Aloe Vera Aromatherapy Gel.

Add 50 drops of the "Anti-Hypertension Blend" to one cup (8 oz or 250 ml) of aloe vera gel to create a non-greasy, healing moisturizer.

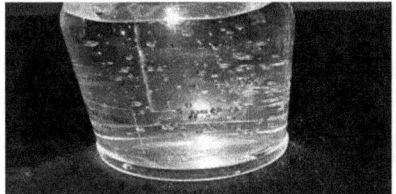

Body Massage Oil.

Add 50 drops (2.5 ml or ½ teaspoons) of the "Anti-Hypertension Blend" to one cup (8 oz or 250 ml) of sweet almond oil or sunflower oil or any other carrier oil to create a healing body massage oil.

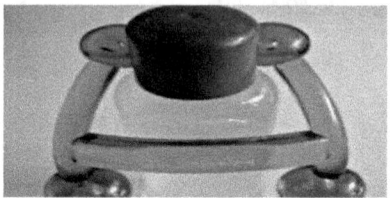

Personal Perfume.

Put 10 ml jojoba in a bottle and add 60 drops of the "Anti-Hypertension Blend" followed by 10 ml of 99% alcohol isopropyl in a spray bottle to make your pressure lowering perfume.

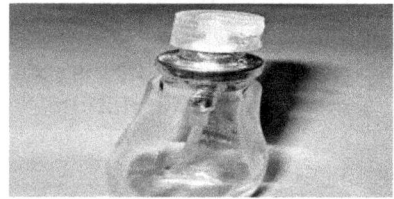

Hair Oil.

Add 50 drops (2.5 ml or ½ teaspoons) of the "Anti-Hypertension Blend" to 1 cup (8 oz or 250 ml) of sweet almond oil or sunflower oil or any other carrier oil to create a hair oil that can also be used for therapeutic scalp massages.

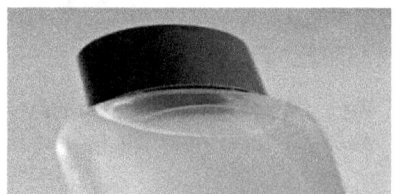

Inhalation Balls.

Add 6 drops of the "Anti-Hypertension Blend" to your handkerchief or a cotton ball and sniff it throughout the day whenever you begin to feel tense or you check your blood pressure and find it is high.

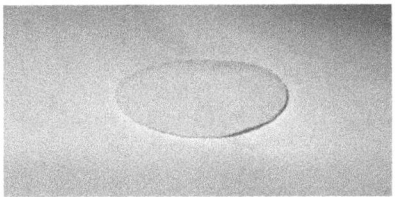

Room Fragrance.

Add 24 drops of the "Anti-Hypertension Blend" to your diffuser. If your diffuser comes with instructions, use the number of drops recommended by the manufacturer.

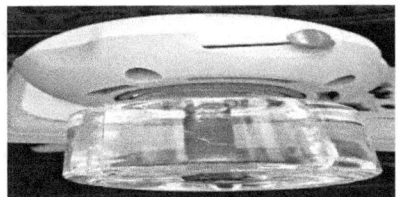

Room Scent.

Add 12 drops of the "Anti-Hypertension Blend" to ¼ cup (2 oz or 60 ml) of water, place it on an oil warmer and light the candle to scatter the healing scent.

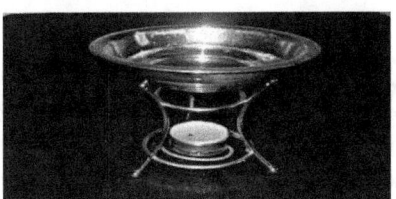

Light Bulb Scent.

Drop 3 drops of the "Anti-Hypertension Blend" to a light bulb when the light is switched off, switch it on to illuminate and scent your room.

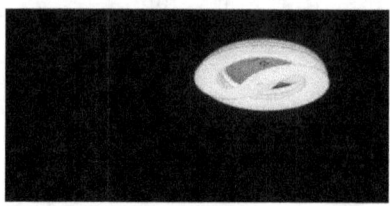

Aroma Ring Scent.

Add 5 drops of the "Anti-Hypertension Blend" to an aroma oil ring, place it on top of your lamp bulb, light the lamp and experience therapeutic lighting.

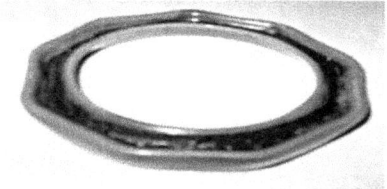

Car Diffuser.

Add the "Anti-Hypertension Blend" to your car's diffuser according to the manufacturer's instructions and let the healing scent envelope you as you drive.

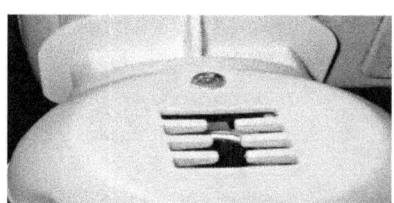

* * * * *

5

LIFESTYLE MODIFICATIONS

Lifestyle modifications that can help lower high blood pressure include:

1.

Exercise Regularly

Regular exercise is very important for regulating blood pressure since it:

1. Helps relax the artery walls and lower blood pressure

2. Helps reduce excess body weight which contributes to high blood pressure

3. Helps manage stress which also raises the blood pressure as it is an effective relaxation technique.

Therefore, regardless of whether you have prehypertension (BP 120/80 to 139/89) or you have full blown hypertension, aim to exercise for 30 to 60 minutes four days a week since studies have shown that it can reduce blood pressure in just a few weeks.

As you do so, space the exercise sessions evenly throughout the week and do not cram them into the weekends.

***

2.

Loose Excess Weight

Losing weight is vital for lowering blood pressure since blood pressure usually rises as a person's weight increases and drops when they lose the excess weight. In addition, the excess weight places extra pressure on the heart and blood vessels.

This weight loss does not have to be dramatic for it to be beneficial since losing just 10 lbs (4.5 kg) or even 5 to 10% of the body weight can lower blood pressure and help the medications prescribed to treat it work more effectively.

***

3.

Limit Alcohol Intake

Drinking one alcoholic drink a day for women and men over 65 years old and two alcoholic drinks a day for men younger than 65 years can lower your blood pressure by 2 to 4 mmHg.

Therefore limit your alcohol intake since this protective effect is lost if one exceeds these daily limits. In addition, drinking more than moderate amounts of alcohol can elevate blood pressure rise and render the medications used to treat it less effective.

NB One alcoholic drink is 12 oz (360 ml) of beer or 5 oz (150 ml) of wine or 1.5 oz (45 ml) of 80 proof liquor.

***

4.

Manage Stress

Emotional stress and anxiety can raise blood pressure due to the stress hormones produced during the body's stress reaction. Chronic stress can therefore cause poorly controlled blood pressure which can increase a person's risk of developing hypertension complications.

Therefore , learn effective relaxation techniques so that you can manage stress effectively.

Research has also shown that persons with mild hypertension who practiced ancient relaxation techniques like yoga, qigong and tai chi which combine gentle body movements and controlled breathing daily for between two and three months, were able to lower their blood pressure.

Therefore incorporate these exercises into your lifestyle or the Christian alternative of breathing rhythmically as you do the following exercises:

1. **Neck Stretch** - Stand with your feet shoulder width apart and your chin on your chest. Rotate your head once clockwise. Return chest to chin and rotate it counter clockwise. Do several rotations. Turn your face to the right, look as far back over your shoulder as you can. Hold for a count of 10. Repeat on opposite side.

2. **Chest, Shoulder and Arm Stretch** - Stand with your feet shoulder width apart and your knees slightly bent. Clasp your hands behind your back and push them back as far as you can reach. Push your chest forward as far as it can reach. Hold and return to starting position.

3. **Side Stretch** - Stand straight with your arms raised over your head. Tilt your body to the left side as you stretch your side muscles. Hold. Repeat on the opposite side.

4. **Abs, Glutes and Quads Stretch** - Stand with your feet together. Reach forward with your right arm. Lift your left leg behind you and grasp your left ankle with your left hand. Lift your left thigh as high as you can or until it is parallel to the ground. Repeat on opposite side.

5. **Back Stretch** - Lie on your back and pull both knees to your chest. Release them and lower your knees to the right side and then to the left side. Return knees back to chest.

6. **Hamstring Stretch** - Lie on your back with your legs bent and both feet flat on the floor. Straighten and raise your right leg. Gently pull your right thigh towards your body and hold for a count of 10. Repeat on the opposite side.

***

5.

Stop Smoking

Join a smoking cessation program and stop smoking since nicotine can increase blood pressure by up to 10 mmHg and for up to an hour after the smoking session.

***

6.

Get Adequate Sleep

Get 7-10 hours of sleep every night since it can help you maintain a normal body weight. This is due to the fact that the production of grehlin, an appetite stimulant, by the body decreases during sleep while that of letpin, an appetite suppressant, increases.

***

7.

Foster Spiritual Health

Develop a strong spiritual relationship with God since several studies have shown that people of faith are healthier than non-believers. Other studies have also shown that prayer can reduce the symptoms of some diseases.

Having a relationship with your God can also help you cope with the stress and depression of living with a chronic condition like hypertension and deal with its complications like strokes better.

Therefore, find a Bible preaching Church and practice your faith sincerely since simply going through the motions does not confer any of the faith related health benefits.

* * * * *

6

EXERCISE PLAN

A balanced exercise plan should combine stretching, weight bearing and aerobic exercises.

If you have been leading a sedentary lifestyle, consult your doctor and nutritionist before making changes to your exercise regimen.

In addition, invest in a good pair of sports shoes that will cushion your feet and redistribute your weight evenly as you walk, jog, jump or run.

If as you exercise, you experience any of the following symptoms, stop exercising at once and consult your doctor: chest pain, pressure or tightness, unusual shortness of breath, pain in the jaw, arm, neck or shoulder, palpitations or skipped heart beats, feeling dizzy or fainting, muscle pain that is more severe than just discomfort.

1.

Stretching Exercises

Stretch for at least 10 minutes each morning and evening and in the warm up and cool down periods just before or right after your exercise sessions.

To stretch correctly you should:

1. Not hold your breath as you stretch. Breathe in and out rhythmically.

2. Never bounce into or out of your stretches. Gently move into and out of the various positions.

3. Hold the stretch position for 10 seconds and gradually increase the duration.

4. Be systematic and begin with the legs as you work your way up the body to the neck or vice versa.

5. Stop stretching if you feel any pain but continue if you experience mild discomfort.

The following is a list of exercises that you can do at home to stretch your entire body.

1. Neck Stretch - Stand with your feet shoulder width apart and your chin on your chest. Rotate your head once clockwise. Return chest to chin and rotate it counter clockwise. Do several rotations. Turn your face to the right, look as far back over your shoulder as you can. Hold for a count of 10. Repeat on opposite side.

2. Chest, Shoulder and Arm Stretch - Stand with your feet shoulder width apart and your knees slightly bent. Clasp your hands behind your back and push them back as far as you can reach. Push your chest forward as far as it can reach. Hold and return to starting position.

3. Side Stretch - Stand straight with your arms raised over your head. Tilt your body to the left side as you stretch your side muscles. Hold. Repeat on the opposite side.

4. Abs, Glutes and Quads Stretch - Stand with your feet together. Reach forward with your right arm. Lift your left leg behind you and grasp your left ankle with your left hand. Lift your left thigh as high as you can or until it is parallel to the ground. Repeat on opposite side.

5. Back Stretch - Lie on your back and pull both knees to your chest. Release them and lower your knees to the right side and then to the left side. Return knees back to chest.

6. Hamstring Stretch - Lie on your back with your legs bent and both feet flat on the floor. Straighten and raise your right leg. Gently pull your right thigh towards your body and hold for a count of 10. Repeat on the opposite side.

***

2.

Weight Bearing Exercises

To weight train or strength train correctly you should:

a) Not hold your breath or strain as you train.

b) Not exercise the same muscle groups for two consecutive days.

c) Aim for 3 sets of 10 repetitions each.

The following are exercises that you can do at home to strength train your entire body.

1. Overhead Press - (Works shoulders) Sit on a chair; hold a weight (or a full water bottle) in each hand at shoulder level with palms facing forward. Raise your arms straight up over your head. Lower them to shoulder level.

2. Biceps Curl - (Works biceps) Sit on a chair; hold a weight (or a full water bottle) in each hand palms facing forward. Bend your elbow and lift the weight towards your shoulder. Return to starting position and repeat with the other arm.

3. Triceps Dips - (Works triceps) Sit on the edge of a sturdy chair with your back and shoulders straight. Hold the edge of a chair and bend your elbows to form a right angle as you lower your butt off the seat to the floor. Straighten your arms and press back up to raise your butt back to the seat.

4. Push Ups - (Works deltoids, triceps, pectorals) Lie on floor, palms face down, elbows bent next to shoulders. Push up from floor by straightening elbows and contracting abs so that your body forms a straight line from your head to heel (beginners can rest both knees on floor) Lower yourself to floor by bending elbows. Push back up.

5. Simple Straight Crunches - (Works abs) Lie flat on your back; bend knees while keeping your feet flat on the floor. Place your hands on your thighs. Exhale and lift shoulder blades from the floor as you slide your hands up to your knees. Hold for a count of 10. Return to starting position and repeat.

6. Simple Side Crunches - (Works abs) Lie flat on your back; bend knees while keeping your feet flat on the floor. Place your hands on your right thigh. Exhale and lift shoulder blades from the floor as you slide your hands up to your right knee. Hold for a count of 10. Return to starting position and repeat. Do on opposite side.

7. Advanced Straight Crunches - (Works abs) Lie flat on your back; bend your knees until thighs are perpendicular to floor. Place arms crossed over your chest. Exhale, tighten abs and lift shoulder blades from the floor as you reach towards knees. Hold for a count of 10. Return to starting position and repeat.

8. Advanced Side Crunches - (Works abs) Lie flat on your back; bend your knees until thighs are perpendicular to floor. Place arms crossed over your chest. Exhale, tighten abs and lift shoulder blades from floor as you reach towards right knee. Hold for a count of 10. Return to starting position and repeat. Do on opposite side.

9. Leg Lifts - Lie on your back; legs straight; hands under butt. Lift legs 30 cm from the floor. Hold for a count of 10.

10. Lunge - (Works glutes, hamstrings, quadriceps) Stand with feet shoulder width apart, arms at sides. Take a large step forward with your left leg and ensure your left knee is above your left foot. Lower your body to the floor by bending the right knee until right thigh is parallel to the floor and right knee is close to the ground. Squeeze your glutes as you press back up to your starting position. Repeat on opposite side.

11. Squat - (Works your butt and thighs) Stand with your feet parallel and shoulder width apart. Stretch out your hands in front of you. Keeping your abs and butt tight, bend your knees and slowly lower yourself as though you are sitting. Ensure your knees don't extend past your toes. Hold for a count of 10. As your rise, squeeze your glutes.

12. Calf Raises - (Work your calf muscles) Stand with feet together and arms raised above your head. Lift your heels so that you are standing on the balls of your feet/toes. Stand on your toes for a count of 10.

***

3.

Aerobic Exercises

Aerobic exercises include walking, skipping a rope, jogging (on a treadmill or in the park), cycling or spinning in the gym, swimming, aerobic classes in a gym, sports like tennis and basketball as well as everyday activities like climbing stairs, housework and gardening.

Swimming is a good option especially if you are overweight or obese because it does not put excessive pressure on the joints of the lower limbs.

To reap the most benefits from your aerobic exercise sessions, you should:

1. Exercise for at least 30 min each session

2. Reach your Target Heart Rate (THR) which is calculated by

220 - your age = maximum heart rate (MHR)

MHR x 0.65 = minimum target heart rate (MinTHR)

MHR x 0.80 = maximum target heart rate (MaxTHR)

For example, if you are 40 years old, 220 - 40 years = 180 your maximum heart rate (MHR)

180 (MHR) x 0.65 = 117 your minimum target heart rate (MinTHR)

180 (MHR) x 0.80 = 144 your maximum target heart rate (MaxTHR)

Therefore, as you exercise, you should ensure that your heart rate is between 117 and 144.

To know your heart rate per minute, take your pulse on your wrist or neck for one minute.

The following is a rough guide of target heart rates for different age groups:

If you are 20 years old, your Target Heart Rate (THR) per minute should be 130 - 160

If you are 30 years old, your Target Heart Rate (THR) per minute should be 123 – 152

If you are 40 years old, your Target Heart Rate (THR) per minute should be 117 – 144

If you are 50 years old, your Target Heart Rate (THR) per minute should be 110 – 136

If you are 60 years old, your Target Heart Rate (THR) per minute should be 104 – 128

If you are 70 years old, your Target Heart Rate (THR) per minute should be 97 – 120

If you are 80 years old, your Target Heart Rate (THR) per minute should be 91 – 112

***

Exercise Plan

You can modify this plan to suit your lifestyle and level of activity.

Exercise Activity for Week 1

Day 1

Whole body stretch to warm up

30 min walk at minimum THR

Whole body stretch to cool down

Day 2

Whole body stretch to warm up

10 push ups, 10 triceps dips, 10 crunches

Whole body stretch to cool down

Day 3

Whole body stretch to warm up

30 min walk at minimum THR

Whole body stretch to cool down

Day 4

Whole body stretch to warm up

10 squats, 10 lunges, 10 calf raises, 10 crunches

Whole body stretch to cool down

Day 5

Whole body stretch to warm up

30 min walk at minimum THR

Whole body stretch to cool down

Exercise Activity for week 2

Day 1

Whole body stretch to warm up

30 min walk/ jog at medium THR

Whole body stretch to cool down

Day 2

Whole body stretch to warm up

15 push ups, 15 bicep curls, 15 triceps dips, 15 crunches

Whole body stretch to cool down

Day 3

Whole body stretch to warm up

30 min walk/ jog at medium THR

Whole body stretch to cool down

Day 4

Whole body stretch to warm up

15 squats, 15 lunges, 15 calf raises, 15 crunches

Whole body stretch to cool down

Day 5

Whole body stretch to warm up

30 min walk/ jog at medium THR

Whole body stretch to cool down

Exercise Activity for week 3

Day 1

Whole body stretch to warm up

30 min walk/run maximum THR

Whole body stretch to cool down

Day 2

Whole body stretch to warm up

20 push ups, 20 bicep curls, 20 triceps dips, 20 crunches

Whole body stretch to cool down

Day 3

Whole body stretch to warm up

30 min walk/run maximum THR

Whole body stretch to cool down

Day 4

Whole body stretch to warm up

20 squats, 20 lunges, 20 calf raises, 20 crunches

Whole body stretch to cool down

Day 5

Whole body stretch to warm up

30 min walk/run maximum THR

Whole body stretch to cool down

Exercise Activity for week 4

Day 1

Whole body stretch to warm up

30 min walk/run maximum THR

Whole body stretch to cool down

Day 2

Whole body stretch to warm up

30 push ups, 30 bicep curls, 30 triceps dips, 30 crunches

Whole body stretch to cool down

Day 3

Whole body stretch to warm up

30 min walk/run maximum THR

Whole body stretch to cool down

Day 4

Whole body stretch to warm up

30 push ups, 30 bicep curls, 30 triceps dips, 30 crunches

Whole body stretch to cool down

Day 5

Whole body stretch to warm up

30 min walk/run maximum THR

Whole body stretch to cool down

* * * * *

7

STRESS MANAGEMENT PLAN

Learning and practicing relaxation techniques is a very effective way of managing stress. These relaxation techniques include:

1.

Meditation

Meditation is another effective relaxation technique for coping with stress. To meditate, simply lie down in a quiet place and take several deep breaths. Once your body begins to feel calmer, focus on your inhalation and on the pure oxygen entering your body. As you exhale, envision you whole body relaxing. You can also meditate on Scriptures like **With God all things are possible** (Matthew 19:26) and envisioning your stressful situation resolving miraculously.

***

2.

Abdominal Breathing

Abdominal breathing or deep breathing is one fastest ways of counteracting the body's stress response. It is done by inhaling through your nose until your abdomen rises, holding your breath for a few moments and then exhaling completely through your mouth until your abdomen collapses. This cycle of filling the lungs with air, pausing and then emptying them can be repeated for 15 minutes every day.

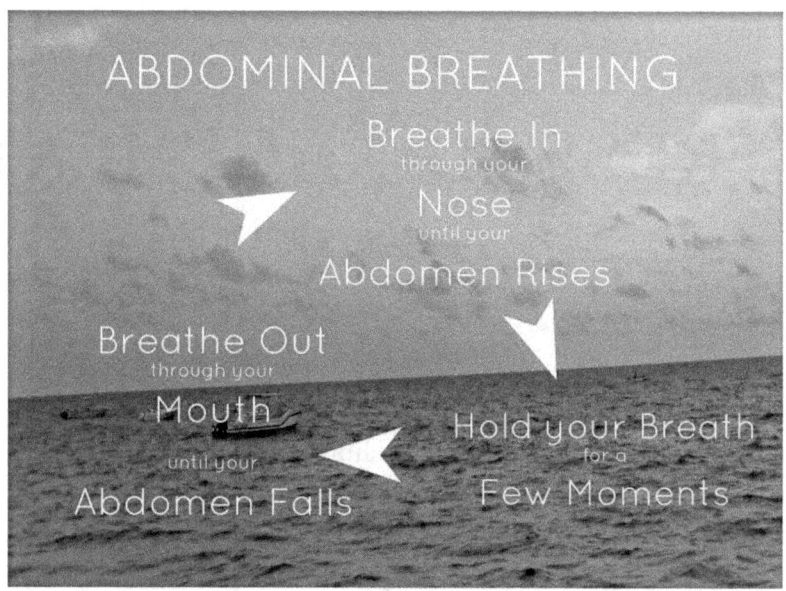

***

3.

Guided Imagery

Guided imagery is another effective relaxation technique. It involves visualizing yourself in a relaxing environment. Therefore close your eyes, take several deep breaths and use your mind's eye to see yourself relaxing on a beach or floating on a cloud or walking through a garden or whichever environment makes you feel relaxed. Use all your senses to immerse yourself in the restful environment by seeing soothing images, smelling appealing scents, hearing calming sounds, tasting and feeling your way through it. After you have enjoyed our visit, bring yourself gently back to reality.

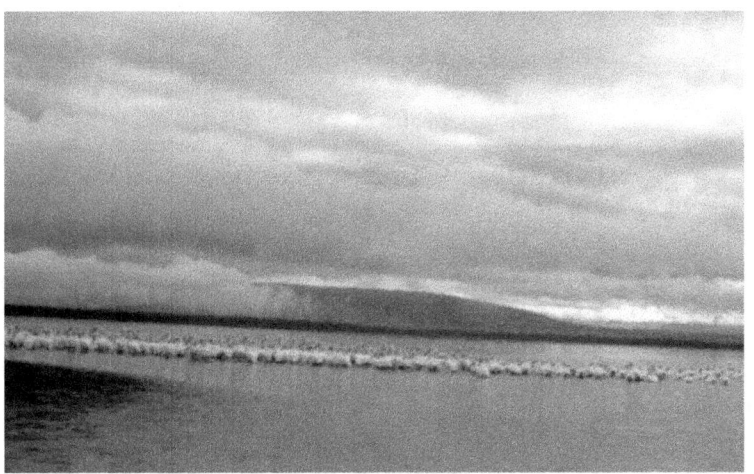

***

4.

Problem Solving Visualization

Visualization can also be used to manage stressful situations. To do this see yourself with your mind's eye in your most stressful situation and then envisioning yourself using various strategies to cope. For example you can imagine yourself dealing with a stressful boss by breathing deeply until you no longer feel distressed by their words or actions.

***

5.

Physical Exercise

When a person is stressed, they tense their muscles. Stretching exercises reduce this muscle tension and help a person feel relaxed.

Aerobic exercises help the body burn circulating stress hormones that contribute to the development of stress related illnesses.

Weight bearing exercises also aid in stress management since they demand concentration and help a person forget their problems.

Therefore engage in regular physical exercises to manage stress.

Relaxing Activities

Other relaxing activities that you can engage in to manage stress include:

1. Journaling since writing down uncensored feelings is a very effective method of catharsis. It is doubly effective when combined with writing lists of things you are thankful for.

2. Listening to calming music.

3. Engaging in hobbies that complement their main job

4. Helping less fortunate members of your society like visiting the sick in hospitals since this takes your mind off your problems

5. Drinking soothing herbal teas like chamomile and passionflower.

6. Eating foods which raise serotonin levels like turkey, salmon, chicken, cheese, chocolate, wholegrain bread.

7. Watching comedy since laughter relieves tension.

8. Spending time with your social support system.

***

Stress Management Plan

Stress Management Plan Week 1

Day 1

1. Abdominal breathing

2. Meditation

3. Physical Exercise

4. Watching Comedy

Day 2

1. Abdominal breathing

2. Meditation

3. Drinking herbal teas and eating serotonin rich foods

4. Watching Comedy

Day 3

1. Abdominal breathing

2. Meditation

3. Physical Exercise

4. Watching Comedy

Day 4

1. Abdominal breathing

2. Meditation

3. Drinking herbal teas and eating serotonin rich foods

4. Watching Comedy

Day 5

1. Abdominal breathing

2. Meditation

3. Physical Exercise

4. Watching Comedy

Day 6 and 7

1. Abdominal breathing 2. Meditation 3. Spending time with your social support system

Stress Management Plan Week 2

Day 1

1. Abdominal breathing

2. Guided imagery

3. Physical Exercise

4. Listening to Music

Day 2

1. Abdominal breathing

2. Guided imagery

3. Drinking herbal teas and eating serotonin rich foods

4. Listening to Music

Day 3

1. Abdominal breathing

2. Guided imagery

3. Physical Exercise

4. Listening to Music

Day 4

1. Abdominal breathing

2. Guided imagery

3. Drinking herbal teas and eating serotonin rich foods

4. Listening to Music

Day 5

1. Abdominal breathing

2. Guided imagery

3. Physical Exercise

4. Listening to Music

Day 6 and 7

1. Abdominal breathing 2. Guided imagery 3. Engaging in Complementary Hobbies

Stress Management Plan Week 3

Day 1

1. Abdominal breathing

2. Problem solving visualization

3. Physical Exercise

4. Journaling and writing gratitude lists

Day 2

1. Abdominal breathing

2. Problem solving visualization

3. Drinking herbal teas and eating serotonin rich foods

4. Journaling and writing gratitude lists

Day 3

1. Abdominal breathing

2. Problem Solving Visualization

3. Physical Exercise

4. Journaling and writing gratitude lists

Day 4

1. Abdominal breathing

2. Problem Solving Visualization

3. Drinking herbal teas and eating serotonin rich foods

4. Journaling and writing gratitude lists

Day 5

1. Abdominal breathing

2. Problem Solving Visualization

3. Physical Exercise

4. Journaling and writing gratitude lists

Day 6 and 7

1. Abdominal breathing 2. Problem Solving Visualization 3. Helping the less fortunate

Stress Management Plan Week 4

Day 1

1. Abdominal breathing

2. Meditation or Guided Imagery or Problem Solving Visualization (choose the one that has been most relaxing for you and practice it regularly)

3. Physical exercise

4. Watching Comedy or Listening to Music or Journaling and writing gratitude lists (choose the one that has been most relaxing for you and practice it regularly)

Day 2

1. Abdominal breathing

2. Meditation or Guided Imagery or Problem Solving Visualization (choose the one that has been most relaxing for you and practice it regularly)

3. Drinking herbal teas and eating serotonin rich foods

4. Watching Comedy or Listening to Music or Journaling and writing gratitude lists (choose the one that has been most relaxing for you and practice it regularly)

Day 3

1. Abdominal breathing

2. Meditation or Guided Imagery or Problem Solving Visualization (choose the one that has been most relaxing for you and practice it regularly)

3. Physical exercise

4. Watching Comedy or Listening to Music or Journaling and writing gratitude lists (choose the one that has been most relaxing for you and practice it regularly)

Day 4

1. Abdominal breathing

2. Meditation or Guided Imagery or Problem Solving Visualization (choose the one that has been most relaxing for you and practice it regularly)

3. Drinking herbal teas and eating serotonin rich foods

4. Watching Comedy or Listening to Music or Journaling and writing gratitude lists (choose the one that has been most relaxing for you and practice it regularly)

Day 5

1. Abdominal breathing

2. Meditation or Guided Imagery or Problem Solving Visualization (choose the one that has been most relaxing for you and practice it regularly)

3. Physical exercise

4. Watching Comedy or Listening to Music or Journaling and writing gratitude lists (choose the one that has been most relaxing for you and practice it regularly)

Day 6 and 7

1. Abdominal breathing

2. Meditation or Guided Imagery or Problem Solving Visualization (choose the one that has been most relaxing for you and practice it regularly)

3. Spending time with your social support system or Engaging in complementary hobbies or Helping the less fortunate (choose the one that has been most relaxing for you and practice it regularly)

###

ABOUT THE AUTHOR

Dr. Miriam Kinai is a medical doctor and freelance health writer/blogger.

You can visit her blog at http://www.MyBlogBookClub.com or follow her on twitter at http://twitter.com/AlmasiHealth

Email enquiries to almasihealthcare@yahoo.com with BOOKS as your subject.

HERBS AND SPICES FOR THE COOK, HEALER AND BEAUTICIAN

Herbs and Spices for the Cook, Healer and Beautician uses color pictures and clear explanations to teach you about more than 70 healing herbs and spices.

You will learn about their:

* Therapeutic (healing) uses

* Drug interactions

* Contraindications (when not to use them)

* Cooking tips

* Beauty tips

*****

INTERNATIONAL GOURMET HERB AND SPICE BLENDS

International Gourmet Herb and Spice Blends teaches you how to prepare exotic herb and spice blends from around the world. You will discover the recipes for:

* Barbecue Rub, Cajun, Apple Pie and Pumpkin Pie Spice Mixes from America

* Pudding Spice Mix from Britain

* 5 Spice Mix from China

* Berbere Spice Mix from Ethiopia

* Curry Powder and Garam Masala from India

* Bouquet Garni, Herbs de Provence and Quatre Epices from France

* Herb Mix from Italy

* Jerk Seasoning from Jamaica

* Shichimi Togarashi from Japan

* Pilau Spice Blend from Kenya

* Chili Powder from Mexico

* Baharat Spice Blend from the Middle East

* Ras El Hanout from Morocco

*****

THE QUICK GOURMET CHEF

The Quick Gourmet is an essential culinary skills cookbook which teaches how to make simple, divine dishes.

You will learn how to make:

* Hot Chocolate Mixes and Drinks

* Hot Chai Tea Mixes and Drinks

* Hot Coffee Mixes and Drinks

* Sensational Smoothies

* Non-Dairy Smoothies

* Chocolate Covered Strawberries

* Chocolate Truffles

* Healthy Chicken Salads

* Healthy Tuna Salads

* Savory Salsas

* Herb Butter

* Cheese Dips and Sauces

* Gourmet Sandwiches

* Perfect Hard Boiled Eggs

* A Cheese Board

* Natural Food Color

*****

HOW TO STYLE AND PHOTOGRAPH FOOD

Regardless of whether you are an aspiring food blogger or you want to make money online selling stock photos, How To Style and Photograph Food, uses color pictures and clear explanations to teach you the food photography tips that can help you improve your digital camera photography skills so that you can begin photographing food like a pro.

You will learn:

* The equipment that you need

* How to set up the lighting

* How to prepare the stage

* How to style the food

* How to shoot the food

*****

HOW TO MAKE NATURAL SKIN CARE PRODUCTS VOLUME 1

How To Make Natural Skin Care Products Volume 1 by Dr Miriam Kinai is filled with recipes for making organic bath and body products for normal, sensitive, oily and dry skin types as well as therapeutic products to manage mature skin, prematurely aging skin, cellulite, eczema, psoriasis, ringworms, dandruff, thinning hair, menopausal symptoms, pre-menstrual tension (PMS), painful periods, arthritis, stress, sadness or depression, mental exhaustion and insomnia.

This book also teaches you the best vegetable oils, essential oils, natural butters and herbs to use when making products for different skin types physical conditions. You will learn how to make:

* Bath bombs

* Bath melts

* Bath salts

* Bath teas

* Body butters

* Body lotions

* Body scrubs

* Healing balms and body creams

* Herb infused oils

* Natural soap

How to Make Natural Skin Care Products Volume 1 will leave you with a clear understanding of how to make bath and beauty products to use in your home or to give as gifts or to sell and make money.

*****

ORGANIC SKIN CARE PRODUCT INGREDIENTS

Organic Skin Care Product Ingredients teaches you about the different natural substances that can be used to create natural bath and beauty products to use in your home or to give as gifts to your loved ones or to sell and make money.

You will learn about:

* Natural butters

* Natural clays

* Natural colorants

* Natural exfoliants

* Natural fragrances

* Natural oils

* Natural preservatives

*****

THE ESSENTIALS OF AROMATHERAPY ESSENTIAL OILS

The Essentials of Aromatherapy Essential Oils by Dr Miriam Kinai teaches you how to use aromatherapy oils to improve your physical, mental and emotional well being.

The author's experience as a medical doctor and clinical aromatherapy practitioner have enabled her to write a highly informative guide for those who want to utilize the healing benefits of these natural plant essences.

You will discover:

* The safety information and therapeutic uses of 18 essential oils

* How to blend essential oils

* The characteristics and uses of 14 carrier oils

* How to Dilute Essential Oils with Carrier Oils

* How to Use Essential Oils

* Cautionary Measures when using Essential Oils

* Numerous Essential Oil Recipes for bath products as well as skin care and hair care products

The Essentials of Aromatherapy Essential Oils will leave you with a clear understanding of how you can safely use aromatherapy essential oils to heal yourself naturally.

*****

CARRIER OILS GUIDE

Carrier Oils Guide teaches you the characteristics, health benefits and uses of commonly used carrier oils. You will learn about:

* Apricot Kernel Oil

* Avocado Oil

* Borage Seed Oil

* Calendula Oil

* Carrot Seed Oil

* Castor Oil

* Evening Primrose Oil

* Fractionated Coconut Oil

* Jojoba

* Olive Oil

* Rosehip Oil

* Sunflower Oil

* Sweet Almond Oil

* Virgin Coconut Oil

* Useful formulas for Diluting Essential Oils with Carrier Oils

*****

MEDICAL AROMATHERAPY FOR HEALTH PROFESSIONALS

Medical Aromatherapy for Healthcare Professionals by Dr Miriam Kinai teaches you how to use essential oils to treat physical diseases and emotional disorders.

The author's experience as a medical doctor and clinical aromatherapy practitioner have enabled her to write a highly informative guide for those who want to utilize the healing benefits of these natural plant essences.

You will discover how to use essential oils to:

* Treat skin diseases like acne, eczema and psoriasis

* Treat other physical diseases like high blood pressure, arthritis, coughs and colds

* Manage mental and emotional conditions like anxiety, depression, anger and stress

* Relieve the symptoms of menopause and premenstrual tension

* Lessen insomnia and impotence

Medical Aromatherapy for Healthcare Professionals is therefore an essential resource for holistic healthcare practitioners like massage therapists, naturopaths and herbalists.

It is also a useful resource for conventional medicine healthcare providers like physicians and nurses who want to begin practicing integrative medicine and for patients who want to improve their health naturally by using aromatherapy oils.

*****

AROMATHERAPY COURSE

Aromatherapy Course by Dr Miriam Kinai tutors you on how to use essential oils to improve your physical, mental and emotional well being.

The author's experience as a medical doctor and clinical aromatherapy practitioner have enabled her to create a highly informative course on how to use these natural plant essences.

You will learn:

* The safety information and therapeutic uses of essential oils like clary sage, eucalyptus, geranium, grapefruit, lavender, lemon, lemongrass, marjoram, orange (sweet), patchouli, peppermint, Roman chamomile, rose, rosemary, sandalwood, spearmint, tea tree and ylang ylang.

* The safety information and therapeutic uses of carrier oils like apricot kernel oil, avocado oil, borage seed oil, calendula oil, carrot seed oil, castor oil, evening primrose oil, fractionated coconut oil, jojoba, olive oil, rosehip oil, sunflower oil, sweet almond oil and virgin coconut oil.

* How to blend essential oils

* How to dilute essential oils with carrier oils

* How to administer essential oils

* How to make natural healing products from numerous aromatherapy recipes

* How to utilize the healing benefits of essentials oils even if you do not have prior training in aromatherapy

The Aromatherapy Course will leave you with a clear understanding of how you can heal yourself and your family naturally by using essentials oils on your body and in your home.

*****

DEALING WITH DEPRESSION NATURALLY

Dealing with Depression Naturally presents a holistic approach to managing depression with natural antidepressants. You will learn how to treat depression with:

* Aromatherapy

* Art therapy

* Christian Biblical principles

* Chromotherapy

* Diet therapy

* Eco-therapy

* Herbal therapy

* Home decor therapy

* Music therapy

* Phototherapy

* Exercise therapy

* Self-Psychotherapy

* Social therapy

* Talk therapy

* Vitamin therapy

* Writing therapy

*****

CHRISTIAN LIFE COACHING HANDBOOK

Christian Life Coaching Handbook offers a Biblical approach to managing different aspects of life.

You will learn:

* Christian anger management

* Christian conflict resolution

* Christian depression treatment

* Christian goal setting

* Christian marital stress management

* Christian stress management

* How to assert yourself

* How to defeat fear

* How to love yourself

* How to overcome shyness

* How to resist temptation

* How to stop being a people pleaser

*****

CHRISTIAN PERSONAL FINANCE

Christian Personal Finance teaches Biblical principles of money management.

You will learn:

* Christian financial stress management from people who were dealing with money stress like the Acts 3 beggar or credit issues like the widow in second Kings.

* Biblical prosperity principles from wealthy men and women of God like Isaac and the Proverbs 31 woman.

* Bible verses to use as spiritual warfare prayers and as Christian finance affirmations and Christian money meditations.

*****

ANTHOLOGY OF CHRISTIAN BIBLE SERMONS

Anthology of Christian Bible Sermons is a compilation of more than 20 Biblical rhema teachings which include:

* A New Christmas Message

* A New Easter Message

* Are You A Flamboyant Fig Tree Christian?

* Biblical Lessons for Purim from Queen Esther

* Can God Help Me If I Am Surrounded By Enemies?

* How Badly Do You Really Want It?

* Seed Words And The Powerful Tongue

* Spiritual AIDS

* The Three Levels Of Getting Lost

* Why Does God Allow Suffering?

* Your Life Is Your Ministry And Your Storm Is Your Message

* A Perfect God, Imperfect People, and Perfect Plans

* We Are Not Ignorant of His Devices

* How to Prepare for a Dangerous Journey

* Yes, God Can

* How to Serve the Body of Christ

* Conduits of God

* Go Back? Stand Still? Move Forward? Drown?

*****

CHRISTIAN SPIRITUAL WARFARE

Christian Spiritual Warfare teaches you the awesome Bible verses you can use as spiritual warfare prayers, Christian affirmations and in your Christian meditation sessions as you fight your spiritual battles.

You will learn how to fight for the following with Bible verses:

* Marriage * Children * Health

* Christian Faith * Christian Ministry

* Country

* Finances * Job * Business

* Peace of Mind * Restoration * Self Esteem * Self Love

You will also learn how to fight against the following with Bible verses:

* Addiction * Temptation

* Being Single * Infertility

* Opposition * Oppression

* Worry * Fear

* Feelings of Condemnation * Confusion

* Danger * Death * Despair * Discouragement

* Impatience * Insomnia * Laziness * Loneliness

* Poverty * Pride * Sadness

* Vengeance * Weakness

* A Foul Mouth * Lying

*****

DARK SKIN DERMATOLOGY COLOR ATLAS

Dark Skin Dermatology Color Atlas is filled with clear explanations and color photos of skin, hair, and nail diseases affecting people with skin of color or Fitzpatrick skin types IV, V, and VI.

Topics covered include Acne Vulgaris, Alopecia Areata, Anal Warts, Angioedema, Aphthous Ulcers, Atopic Dermatitis, Blastomycosis, Blister Beetle Dermatitis or Nairobi Fly Dermatitis, Cellulitis, Chronic Ulcers, Confetti Hypopigmentation, Cutaneous T Cell Lymphoma, Cutaneous Tuberculosis, Dermatitis Artefacta, Erythema Nodosum,

Exfoliative Erythroderma, Gianotti Crosti Syndrome, Hand Dermatitis, Hemangioma, Herpes Zoster, Ichthyosis, Ingrown Toenails, Irritant Contact Dermatitis, Kaposi Sarcoma, Keloids, Keratoderma Blenorrhagica, Klippel Trenaunay Weber Syndrome, Leishmaniasis, Leprosy, Leukonychia, Lichen Nitidus, Lichen Planus,

Lichenoid Drug Eruption, Linear Epidermal Nevus, Linear IgA Dermatosis (LAD), Lipodermatosclerosis, Lymphangioma Circumscriptum, Miliaria, Molluscum Contagiosum, Neurofibromatosis, Nickel Dermatitis, Onychomadesis, Onychomycosis, Palmoplantar Eccrine Hidradenitis, Papular Pruritic Eruption (PPE), Paronychia, Pellagra, Pemphigus Foliaceous,

Pemphigus Vulgaris, Piebaldism, Pityriasis Rosea, Pityriasis Rubra Pilaris, Plantar Hyperkeratosis, Plantar Warts, Poikiloderma, Postinflammatory Hyperpigmentation and Hypopigmentation, Post Topical Steroids Hypopigmentation, Psoriasis, Pyogenic Granuloma or Lobular Capillary Hemangioma, Scabies, Seborrheic Dermatitis, Steven Johnson Syndrome (SJS) and Toxic Epidermal Necrolysis (TEN),

Sunburn, Systemic Sclerosis, Tinea Capitis, Tinea Pedis, Tinea Versicolor, Traction Alopecia, Urticaria, Vasculitis, Vitiligo, and Xanthelasma.

*****